ISDN: 978-1467982801

First Printing Date: 10-05-05
Second Printing Date:
Cover Design: Smash Graphics
Editing: Creative Persuasion
Printed in the United States of America

website: www.resolutions.bz
Blogs: www.resolutionsblog.com
        www.gregryanfitness.com

  You Tube Linked in

About the Author

At age 45, Greg Ryan's career began thirty years ago as a professional fitness trainer. In 1986 he won his first of two Michigan bodybuilding championships. He won his second title in 1988. In 1990 he moved to Los Angeles California, where his knowledge enthusiasm and skill attracted the attention of fitness guru Kathy Smith.

During this time Greg ran one of the largest personal training businesses in LA. Attracting numerous high profile movies stars such as Brooke Shields, Bridget Fonda, Connie Sellecca and many more. Greg built a reputation for exercise and behavior change and in the fall of 1992 appeared on the Today Show and Good Morning America.

In 1994 Greg returned to college to further his knowledge in Physical Therapy. During this time Greg's gift of motivating individuals led him to production of his own television segment on FOX TV.

1997 Greg relocated to Louisville Kentucky were he built and operated a private clinic specializing in obesity and diabetic weight loss programs.

Numerous bodybuilding titles, movie star clients, over a dozen authored books and counting; this has made him one of the most experienced and sought after experts in the business. Today Greg has acquired almost a hundred thousand hours of personal training to go with his well rounded career.

Why should you read this book?

Whether coming from a close friend, the nightly news or a letter in the mail, it's difficult to face the truth. Hearing it can really cut to the core and test the very existence of our being. Today, fitness books are filled with advertisements, pill pushers and unrealistic programs that give people false hope. My intention in this book is to give you real hope and with that you'll get straight talk.

It is not my goal to come across in a harsh way, but understand I don't know how else to say what I've observed over the last twenty years. Americans have been HAD because you have not received the truth about what it really takes to be fit and to stay healthy.

Quick fixes abound, but the truth is **there are no quick fixes** that really work...or that last.

It is my responsibility as a fitness professional to provide you with the facts. It is my hope that you read this book with an open mind and that you comprehend that if you don't do something about your health today, tomorrow you may say,

"If only I had known."

Live, Love and Laugh

While these words may be hard to swallow, remember life is still a playground. Inside we are kids who want to play with the toys, enjoy close friendships, and leave some kind of mark before we part this world.

My advice is to take your health seriously, but don't forget to; LIVE like there's no tomorrow, LOVE people for whom they are and LAUGH all the way to heaven's gates.

Preface

Years ago there was a game show called, *"Truth or Consequences."* The contestants were asked silly questions and had to answer correctly before the buzzer sounded. If they did not give the "Truth," they had to face the "Consequences" — usually a funny and embarrassing stunt.

In reality, sometimes it is hard to face the truth, especially when it has to do with your health. You can either choose to face the situation on your terms or inevitably face the consequences on life's terms. If you choose, then you have home field advantage; the choices may not be any easier, but they are more manageable since you're in control of the decisions.

Truth or Consequences is not about fantasy fitness programs. It is about your attitude toward exercise and eating. It's about whether you are going to pay a price ultimately — in your wallet or in your body.

In *Truth or Consequences* you must: 1) face the seriousness of your health and the consequences of your actions, 2) learn what your motives are, and 3) decide how to direct your long-range desires toward better fitness.

This book helps you face the reality before life deals out the consequences. If you don't exercise at all or are motivated on your current program, you need to figure out why. This book does not offer pipe dreams and "get fit quick," answers to common questions. However, it will help you realize what those answers are and point you in the right direction.

Acknowledgement

This book is dedicated to people who have not been afraid to, tell me the truth, hold me to my goals, and encourage me when I needed it the most. Thank you for the honesty and support. Special thanks to God for the timing of it all.

Contents

Part Four: What do I have to do to get out of denial?

Part Five: How do I motivate myself?

Part Six: What reasons should I start?

For twenty years I have consistently sustained a high degree of motivation. I miss exercising when I don't do it and more importantly, I don't feel as healthy or as good about myself emotionally.

Greg Ryan

Part One
What If?

Pride fuels the engine of denial which runs the car of laziness!

Greg Ryan

Introduction

Dad, we need to talk. I know you don't want to talk about it, nor do I think you'll listen, but in all fairness to mom, you need to decide what you want her (us) to do. If it were just all that simple!

By far the most stubborn person I have ever met. Only twice have I ever seen him in this state and I'm not sure it will be the same way again; humbled. This is the third time in as many years he's been in the hospital for the same reason; failing to take the blood pressure medication.

Why dad, why haven't you taken your medication like the doctor said? "If I'm feeling ok why do I need it?" Old school thinking I guess, but the dumbest thing I've every heard. If he won't take his BP medication how in the world will mom and I get him to sign the papers?

The man is as prideful as he is full of fear. Oh, he'll never ever admit it, but losing control or hearing the truth is more of a death wish than missing a few pills here and there.

Dad we need to talk. It's not fair for mom to not know what you would want her to do in case an emergency decision needs to be made. It's not fair for her to go at it alone.

If I were you I would be scared too, I would be terrified of the sight and chance that my life slowly coming to an end, but for once, for just this time dad allow her to do the right thing. Please, I beg of you, don't be stubborn sign the papers. It doesn't mean you're giving up it just allows others to make hard decisions when you may not be capable of making them. The consequences are just too great, dad.

Maybe he's thinking he's got more time.

1

More Money Than Time

If only I had known my time was up?

Yesterday I had all the time in the world, today I'm not so sure. Growing up, I thought life would go on forever – today every moment passes bye in the blink of an eye and tomorrow is only a wish away.

I'm a *"Baby Boomer,"* don't much like the label, but I am getting older and it's just a fact. The question I keep asking myself is, *"Am I doing enough for my health?"* Like many, I think tomorrow will always be there. My heart tells me to do *something,* yet I do nothing.

I have lived most of my life trying to make enough *money* to live comfortably in the confines of my home, lifestyle and family. It never dawned on me to make enough *time* to take care of my health.

I'm better off financially today, yet time is growing shorter, and I can't leverage days or minutes. In my youth I felt invincible; today I'm feeling the inevitable.

Close to Home

I look at my father and see that he's losing the fight. Now in his eighty's, everyday is a struggle of what was, what might have been and now what has become of him. Dad has more money than time and whether he likes it or not life is closing in on him. I wish he would realize that his struggles lie more in the head than in the body.

I admire, but I don't want to experience his regrets. Being my dad and seeing him struggle hits home a lot more. Unfortunately, sometimes the closer to the heart the situation occurs the more you will take it too heart.

I find myself asking, *"If I don't take the time too take care of me now, then will my money out last my time?"*

If Only

If only you knew when you were going to die, would you really want to know? Would you do anything differently when you found out? If you had a choice of living longer or living a better quality of life, which would you choose, longer or better?

People often think, *"if only"* they had known they were going to die, or had to have the surgery they would have done things much different.

IF ONLY...I had known this was going to happen; maybe I would have stopped smoking, laid off a few hamburgers and fries. IF ONLY...I would have taken the stairs, rode my bike, had a medical check up more often; just not stressed so much about life.

What if you could actively change the outcome of your life by eating better and getting daily exercise?

What if had more energy, less pain, and a better attitude toward aging?

What if you approached life with more confidence, rather than dreading the day?

"If only you had known."

I didn't have much time to pack; matter of fact, I'm still wearing the same clothes I put on that morning. I met all three of them on the way up. They said they would hitch a ride, but they weren't sure they would be welcome where I was going.

It was scary to learn how much they knew. Had I met them at some restaurant? Did I see them at the doctor's office? I know, maybe it was the golf course or at a party? I just couldn't put my finger on how I knew these guys until now.

It's pretty nice here — peaceful, always something to do, good conversation. However, I sure miss my family. I wish I hadn't bailed on them, <u>but how would I have known</u>?

The three of them said they warned me many times. How? When? Where? I wondered. I thought I read all the right stuff and sought advice from the right people. I even participated at times.

Lazy *was probably the one I got along with the best. He was the only transparent one of the three. Seeing us together you might have thought we were twins; we were so much alike.*

*The other two were more reserved, but I realized quickly they were stubborn old souls with rough edges—two of the biggest know-it-alls I had ever met. They called themselves **Denial and Pride.***

As I crossed that line, I will never forget what they said, "If only you had known."

The truth is you'll leave anytime, for any reason; how you decide to live those days before you do is up to you. You can choose a path with achy joints, low energy levels, high stress, and poor eating habits or choose a different one.

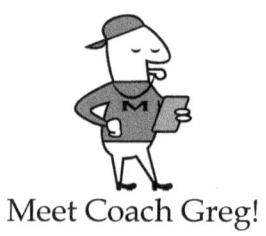

Meet Coach Greg!

2
Reality Bites

Get the facts first!

The Silent Treatment

The health of America is going to get worse before it gets better. Diabetes, obesity, osteoporosis, heart disease—are all at epidemic levels. Today there are more obese people than those just over weight. And for the first time in history kids today are projected not to live as long as there parents will.

The *only* way for America to get better is for YOU to be personally responsible, change the attitude you have toward exercise and be held accountable.

The silent threesome of **denial, pride, and lazy** has been muted by the fantasy fitness land programs promises immediate results. This silent treatment is killing you from the INSIDE OUT. Most of you think that by ignoring the problem the body will miraculously get better. Oh, if only you knew?

The Buck Stops Where?

In the *"good years,"* more money, more marketing and *more-for-me* attitudes enabled us to focus on making the big bucks. It allowed us to put off worrying about the long term; the accent is on NOW. Unfortunately the fiscal wealth we accumulated in the past is now being drained by our physical healthcare costs.

Obesity alone cost our country more than any of our military costs around the world in a single year?

The responsibility falls with some of the big corporations, insurance companies and hospital groups, but at the end of the day the truth of the matter is, **the buck stops with YOU.**

The reality of the situation bites; however the solution is not to igore it, but address it head on. Many of you have either given up on yourself or just flat out are living in denial; either way the choice is still yours. The fact of the matter is there is still hope for America and there is still hope for you, too.

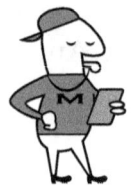

You will only start changing your attitude toward exercise when the consequences start to become the reality.

Coach Greg

Part One: What if you knew your health was bad?

3   Face the Music – *How to deal with the facts about your health!*

3
Facing the Music

Dealing with the Facts

What if you knew that you would face some sort of health problem sooner rather than later if you didn't get some exercise?

What if your kids end up in the same shape you're in right now? Is that fair to them?

What if tomorrow a stroke, heart attack, or cancer struck your life or one you love?

Our country is now *facing the music* for past actions; the problem is it's not on your terms. It is expected that millions will have weak bones, get diabetes, become obese, and die of heart disease in the next ten years. Will you be one of them? Will your children be apart of the crisis?

There are no guarantees that healthy living will add one more day to your life, but *what if* it could? At the very least, *what if* the quality of your life was better?

First thing, face the music by embracing the reality. Accepting the facts does not mean you're admitting defeat, it means you are starting a foundation to build off of.

If you need a health check up, get it. Not knowing is worse than getting the truth. If you need help, then ask. Two good heads work better together than one bad heart.

In my father's eyes

"If only I had known this was going to happen?" That's what my father said last year after suffering a heart attack. A man who showed no fear, never sweated under pressure or complained about anything, laid in a hospital bed acting as a scared little boy who had just lost his mother in a grocery store.

"If only I had known, I would have taken my blood pressure medicine, eaten less fried stuff, and maybe I would have walked a little more," he whispered.

Denying the situation, being prideful by not taking his medication and even being lazy at times almost got the best of my father that day; the next time he may not be so blessed. Next time YOU may not be either!

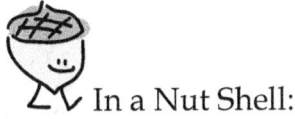 In a Nut Shell:

Life sometimes has a way of giving us slight hints or sometimes shocking wake-up calls. The question is, *"Will you answer the call?"*

You may not be able to change the ultimate outcome, but you sure can change how you feel by getting daily exercise and betting foods than you are now. What would your life be like if you felt better, had more energy and lowered your stress levels? Can you imagine?

There are no guarantees that exercise and eating will prolong death or ward off a disease. The bottom line; *denying* your health is a losing cause, entertaining *pride* is a waste of energy and being *lazy* is no excuse for anything. In the end, you and you alone will decide to accept the truth or deal with the consequences. Why take that chance, why not start now?

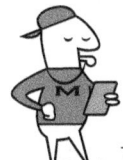 From the coach's box:

- Realize you are not an exception. Bad health can affect anyone at anytime.

- Recognize that denial, pride and laziness are just fictional characters in your head. And they all are born out of FEAR.

- Facing the consequences on your terms is a lot more rewarding than facing the unexpected. A good offense is the best attitude to have.

- Exercise and eating right can be a positive, rewarding and fun thing in anyone's life. It comes down to your attitude.

Part Two
Why Now?

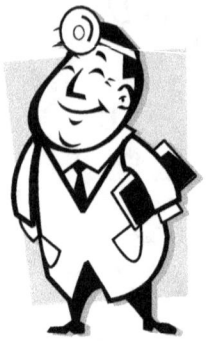

"Pay me now or pay me later!"

4
Pay Now or Pay Later!

Why have I allowed myself to get into this kind of shape?

With life comes responsibility and with decisions comes consequences. Sooner or later you will be in front of the piper, you can pay him now or you can pay later. If you wait you will pay a lot of interest in the form of pain and/or inconvenience, no getting around that. Just look at our economy, the payment has come due plus interest.

The keys to success lie in overcoming these three emotions: *denial, pride and laziness.*

Death by Denial

Has denial ever made you think things like;

"My diet is not that bad.""

A few trips to the fast food joint once in awhile won't hurt."

"My blood pressure is fine, It wouldn't hurt if I skipped a day of taking my medication."

"My New Year's resolution is to get in better shape."

"Why have I let myself get this out of shape?

or "It won't happen to me...no way!"

Unfortunately, it's what's not seen that's killing you. Your insides are getting eaten up ever so slowly, both physically and emotionally. Physically your health has suffering with lack of activity, and poor eating habits. Emotionally, by not facing the facts your self-esteem suffers; leading to a slow and painful death of the soul if not a physical one in the end.

Society is so concerned with makeover television shows that we have been caught off guard with silent killers such as; heart disease, diabetes and obesity.

We overlook the long-term consequence of our behaviors. We see things going on around us, but we continue to put off exercise and eating better for another day. Denial is a form of *pride*.

Pride before the fall

Ever find yourself saying or thinking,

"If I cannot do it on my own, then I will not do it at all."

"Just the very fact of having to take better care of me, irritates me."

"I'll put off my check up until next fall."

First let me say there are two different ways of looking at pride; taking pride or stubborn pride.

My father would say, *"Son never let them see you sweat or they may think you're weak."*

Other times he would encourage me to, *"take pride"* in my work or in other words, care.

Both perspectives are forms of pride; one is a positive and up lifting, while the other is ego and low self esteem.

The positive side of pride is when you so call *"take pride"* in something; when you feel good about a project, event or objective.

The other side (negative) of pride reveals feelings of stubbornness, envy, and even resentment. I believe pride cost thousands of lives every year by promoting inactivity and depression.

Why be so stubborn? Why care what others feel, it's your health? Why such an ego that's so paralyzing you don't do anything? If you think about it, this way of thinking is really down right stupid.

Lazy is what lazy does

"I'll start tomorrow on an exercise program."

Exercise and eating healthy takes discipline, for some that's too much to ask. If that's you, you may be missing out on a really wonderful healthy quality filled life. But, maybe that's not even enough motivation for you?

Why is America the fattest nation in the world? Pure laziness! It's just that simple. If you think a pill, surgery or wishful thinking is going to replace hard work you have been HAD by the media. It takes consistent work, even hard work at times.

Learned Helplessness

Learned helplessness is basically when someone or society does something for you when you are fully capable of doing it yourself. Over time this behavior becomes a feeling of helplessness even entitlement. Something that was meant for good can even be turned into learned helplessness...ie the welfare system.

Its not the fault of the system, but those who have taken advantage of it.

Technology

Rick Pitino one of my favorite basketball coaches said once,

"Technology is ruining our athletes; they are more concerned with pleasing their friends on "Face Book" and reading their text messages after a game rather than just playing the game for themselves or the love of it."

Email systems have disconnected people and genuine communication has suffered. Text messaging has almost dismantled the spelling and English system. People have become addicted to technology and what high it gives them.

Recently our town suffered an ice storm and my email was down for a week; I truly felt uncomfortable and out of whack, how sad? I won't even go into the affects of the video games.

Protectionism

Protectionism is a word that describes how kids and some adults are treated these days.

I grew up on a farm and rarely did I ever get sick. One of the neighbor boys always seemed to have a cold. We never understood why his mother would always make him dress in the summer like it was the dead of winter. Another neighbor boy is thirty- five years old now and still lives with his parents.

My nephew's school teacher is getting sued by the parents of another child for calling him out in front of the others; apparently he spit on one of his class mates. The parents felt their child's discipline was unwarranted and was caused undue stress and embarrassment, so the filed a complaint on the teacher.

Kids these days get away with so much and are given more than the previous generation.

If they fail or fall short of expectations there's someone right there to make an excuse for them or put the blame on something else.

There is a shortage of accountability these days, while society thinks they are protecting people the reality is the opposite, they are weakening the spirit and our survival instincts. The sad thing is learned helplessness, laziness, pride, and denial are all followed up by some sort of price to pay.

Pay now or pay later

The piper will come calling sooner or later, just ask the housing market, car industry or AIG insurance. Financial planners teach people to have an emergency fund for just that, an emergency; if you don't then you will pay a bigger price when you need money for a crisis.

Frankly, you are in major denial if you think you're exempt from someday paying some sort of price either financially or in some form of inconvenience. Denial, pride and laziness can be the end for some, but not for you if you start now.

If paying a price is inevitable and the emergency room (ER) possibly right around the corner, then the big question is, why?

Why are you so resistant toward getting more exercise or eating healthier food? There has to be a reason, not a good one but there is something holding you back.

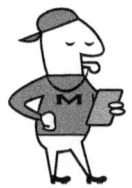

The ER *can be avoided simple by not thinking so much.*

Coach Greg

5
Avoiding the ER!

Why is it so hard for me to start exercising? I know it's good for me. It seems like I have some form of resistance to getting in better shape.

"Exercise Resistance" or **ER** means a conscious or unconscious block against participating in a regular active program. Studies show that some people have barriers built up from past experiences that give them a negative mindset toward exercise and food. In many cases, this prevents a person from starting or following through on an exercise program.

We all have barriers that come in different forms of emotions. Each barrier is usually due to an experience we've had, someone telling us a bold face lie about ourselves in a particular situation or we've just made up some delusional thought on our own.

Resentment

I thought the golden years were supposed to be filled with relaxing things to do, not more activities I usually put off before?

I hate the way I look. In my twenty's I could get away with eating just about anything!

Not wanting to exercise is one thing, but resenting exercise can be paralyzing. Truly, there are only a small percentage of people who like to exercise. And the others do it for a sport or profession. Most people hate the effort, but love the results.

Resentment toward exercise goes much deeper than just not liking the effort; it brings out rebellious attitudes. As we get older, we grow more frustrated and boundaries have to be set, we may even act like a little child at times. We stomp our feet, cross our arms and pout thinking:

"You can't tell me what to do; I'll show you."

The sooner you accept the fact that exercise is going to be a part of your life, the more likely you'll start — the more likely you will continue. Resentment is fueled by being in denial, or full of pride.

Failure

Why should I start exercising? I will not follow through — never have. It will be just another failure.

The only failure is not starting. Success is not measured in numbers. It is measured in your growth through the process. Just because your track record may show some ups and downs has no bearing on your future efforts. Your self-worth is not based on how many times you started an exercise program.

I would rather try and feel good about it efforts even if I didn't succeed rather than having the feeling of regret for never trying. *Fear of failure is just an excuse to never try.*

Perfection

"Why am I not doing this the way I know how? I might as well not do it at all."

If you think for a second that you're going to be perfect sticking to a plan, forget it. The truth is, it will never go the way you want it too. Life brings hurdles, road blocks and forks in the road. If you're frightened about being perfect your intentions are not internal, but for pleasing someone else.

Let me tell you a little secret, no one else really cares if you get a hundred or fail they really only care about themselves. They will forget about you in a day no matter what the out come is. *Perfectionism is an illusion.*

Comparisons

Why do people like Jane look like they do and I have to work so hard? It doesn't seem fair!"

News flash, life isn't fair! For some, it seems effortless to look thin and in good shape.

Some may do the exact workout plan and get totally different results. For you it is a constant trip to the dentist's office, you totally dread it. You need to get beyond fairness.

It's our nature to compare; envy is apart of our emotions. Once you hit a goal there will always be another one. You may even be the type that no matter what you do, it will never be good enough. *Comparing yourself to others and your past is a losing battle, it only brings anger and resentment.*

Expectations

Why is it so hard to balance my fitness goals and lifestyle?

Unless you have such paralyzing health problem there's NO reason not to get some form of exercise. However, you have to be realistic and smart going about it.

If your expectations are too high, you may set yourself up for failure. In some instances exercise resistance (ER) sets in before you even start.

There has to be a happy medium between goals and lifestyles. Set goals that can fit with the demands of your life. Manage time better. *Expectations that are too high are self-defeating before you even start.*

John gets a wake up call

After forty-five years drinking and eating, one or all three of them got to him. The next thing my buddy John knew was he was lying on his back strapped to a heart monitor with a permanent zipper from his belly button to his throat. With a tear in his eye and a cold hand, he said to me, *"If only I had known?"*

"No time to beat yourself up, John," I told him. "You have been spared, learn a lesson and move forward." Later on John told me it was his *pride* that got to him.

One out of three of you will break a bone. Half of you are on the verge of obesity and diabetes. A third of you will suffer a heart attack. Half of you will end up in a nursing home.
And most of you are not living a life filled with confidence, good sleeping patterns, high energy or happiness.

Do the math! Numbers do not lie. You either accept the road less traveled or you face the consequences. It's just that simple. This may resemble a scare tactic, but the bottom line is this is reality.

If you think for one second you are exempt, above reproach, or just relying on luck or faith, think again. Your best defense is a good offense. *Denial, Pride* and *Lazy* will always creep in to make you miserable. They're probably already in your life and you don't see them, but you feel them.

Why now? Resenting the need to exercise is a waste of energy. Never starting because you are afraid of failure is a copout. Striving to exercise to perfection is a bit unrealistic for anyone. Comparing your current condition with how it use to be is a losing battle. And setting expectations so high that your lifestyle prevents you from accomplishing anything is a "bad attitude ready to happen."

Why now? The bottom line, you will pay Doctor Joe eventually if you allow any of the excuses to get to you. Exercising and eating right is the best thing you can do for your mind, body, and your heart. It will take work, but the benefits are priceless.

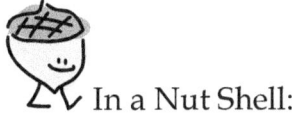 In a Nut Shell:

Let me shoot it to you straight, you're scared. You're fearful of the outcome of a medical test and the reality your situation. You resent the fact that you have not thought about doing anything until now and afraid of not living up to your expectations; in fear of looking bad or it being too late to make a difference.

I have three words for you; get over it!

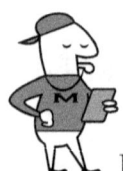 From the coach's box:

➢ Now is as good a time as any to start taking care of you.

➢ Not starting is more of a failure than starting and stopping.

➢ None of us is perfect. If you wait until you think you will be ready, you will never start.

➢ Pride costs! In some cases, it can costs lives.

➢ There is no excuse for laziness.

➢ Exercise Resistance is in your head, not in your stomach.

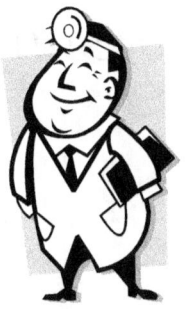

It won't happen to you; go ahead put it off a little longer.

Part Three
When to Start

We are only as strong as our greatest weakness.

Anonymous

6
Why Wait?

Why do New Year's resolutions fail?

Any decision put off is one not taken serious enough. If you have to wait to start on a exercise program or quit a bad eating habit, it's most likely wishful thinking. Goals along the way should be flexible; but once the heartfelt decision is made, there should be no turning back.

I ask you one simple question,

Why Wait?

People wait to start on a program for many reasons:

- I'm too busy.
- Once the kids are back in school.
- After the doctor's checkup.
- I don't feel good today.

The truth, your excuses will never end until you decide to do something about them, NOW!

Have you ever been at a point where you were sick and tired of feeling bad, sleeping restlessly, and having life crashing in on you? If so, then you know what I am about to say is true.

The bottom line is you will only change your habits and attitudes about exercise and eating when — **There are no more options left to explore!**

7

There Are No
More Options Left

One of the most terrifying things to hear is when the doctor says, *"There are no more options, there's nothing we can do."* Can you imagine what life would be like if you had to live thinking that there were no options left, but to die a slow death?

We take life for granted; then all of a sudden something happens to us that resets our thinking.

The Broken Spirit

It seems most people are committed more to an exercise program after some life-changing experience. Unfortunately this has to happen in some cases in order for you to be convinced that something has to be done; it may be a death in the family, a broken bone, and a cancer scare –an event that threatens to take something away from you.

You get to a point of desperation, a broken spirit that says, "Ok, I get the point. What do I have to do? I do not like feeling this way anymore."

In other words, you realize that there are no more options in life, but to move forward on a fitness program and better lifestyle. You have come to accept that the pain of remaining the same is much greater than the pain of changing.

Think back on other times in your life when things were not going so well. Life seemed to force you to slow down and smell the roses a little bit more, didn't it?

Kathy hits rock bottom

Kathy came to me last fall with tears of desperation and frustration in her eyes, *"I cannot take this anymore. I am so miserable inside and out. My heart is tired and heavy. I can't sleep. My joints constantly ache. None of my clothes fit anymore, and I am really afraid of getting diabetes. I have run out of excuses. For the first time in my life I have hit rock bottom. Please help me!"* She pleaded.

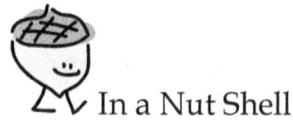 In a Nut Shell

That was the turning point for Kathy. She had run out of excuses. She ran out of self-defeating options. She had reached the bottom and it was a place that she could not stand to be any longer. To this day, Kathy has never looked back.

When will you get to the point of no return? Will your spirit for life have to be broken down so much that you throw up your hands and say, *"I just can't go on like this any longer."* Will the pain have to be so great that it brings you to your knees?

It doesn't have to happen that way if you start taking charge of your life now.

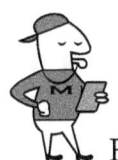 From the coach's box:

> ➤ Do not postpone your decision to exercise and take care of yourself. Waiting only decreases your chance to succeed.

> ➤ Not having enough time to exercise is a bad excuse.

> ➤ Try not to hit rock bottom before you begin to take charge of your life.

Part Four
What's Next?

TIME OUT!

Take a deep breathe, there is still light at the end of the tunnel. Don't give up. Hang in there. Yes, the reality can be burdensome, yet in another way it is refreshing to know where your health stands. Now we take action.

Most people would either give up or start working on the superficial stuff; the only true way to go from a state of denial to a deep desire to be in better shape is from the heart or the **INSIDE OUT.**

8
Denial to Desire

Living in a state of denial can really be a big weight to carry for anyone, no matter what the circumstances are surrounding it. But, what does it mean to be in denial of your health? What are some of the behaviors that are associated with denial?

I know I need to make an appointment for a checkup! But you don't.

I may have a few pounds on me, but I still feel fine.

I walk on the golf course isn't that enough?

I'm going to die sooner or later, why start now on an exercise program?

I don't have enough time.

Ok, I get the point, but……

Where do I go from here? What's next for me?

Deep Desire

Remember those feelings you had back when you wanted your first bicycle or that Barbie doll you made a fit over in front of everyone. Or what about that girl or boy you would have done just about anything to get a date with? You couldn't even think straight, eat or sleep because it occupied every thought. These are all deep desirable aspirations.

Have Hope

Acknowledging the reality of your life does not mean you have to give up on the future; it can mean just the opposite, *"A fresh beginning."*

Many a people have done extraordinary things with nothing but a little bit of hope. Combine that with some faith and a deep desire to feel better, you may be surprised how your life will change, but you have to be open to it.

Open Mind

You have to be open to the idea that exercise and eating better can work for you. You may still recent it but at the same time ask, what if?

You have to accept the fact that life will not hand you a perfect situation, nor that your self-worth is not based upon if you ask for help along the way. We age. Our metabolism slows down, and we are more prone to injuries and illness. However, it does not have to be fatal or depressing if you exercise and eat better.

If the whys are big enough, the how's don't matter!
Niche

The Long-Term Attitude

If you want to go from denial to desire, call on the *"all or nothing attitude."* If you are going to start now, you have to start for good. The reality is you will have good and bad days for the rest of your life. But understand, if you are going to be healthier you have to participate in some form of exercise till the day you die.

This is not a temporary fix to a long-term problem; it is a lifestyle
THE "INSIDE-OUT" APPROACH

It is really important to understand that in order to sustain a healthy lifestyle, you have to develop a positive type of mind set. Sure it looks great and feels great to have a well-shaped body on the outside. However, you will never win the aging battle if you think that all you have to do is work on the outside of the body.

You will have a better chance of feeling better inside and outside if you have a deep desire to be healthy both physically and emotionally first!

When your motives and desires come from the heart or **"INSIDE-OUT"**, then true health begins to grow. And if your physical appearance changes during the process, that is icing on the cake.

Changing from the INSIDE-OUT is a concept or idea, a day-to-day mindset. When your main desire to exercise centers in your heart, it is here you start to live your life with the attitude of

What's next?

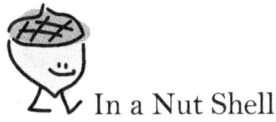 In a Nut Shell

What's next? Only you can answer that question. Being in denial, have too much pride and down right lazy will be your biggest obstacles. And it would be unrealistic to think you will ever be totally rid of them. On the other hand, building a strong desire to stand on your own will be biggest strength against them. When your desire to feel better is so strong, the truth becomes a tool instead of a barrier.

Being in denial, having to much pride and laziness are fictional characters in our minds. While paralyzing, immediate action without compromise tends to scare them away. Waiting to feel better makes no logical sense. Starting right now makes all the sense in the world because the result will be that you feel better.

"If only I had known," you will say.

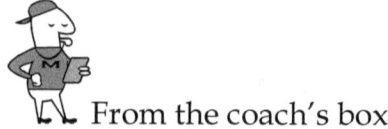 From the coach's box:

➢ The process will be a lot easier with an open-minded, long-term approach to your health.

➢ Most importantly, focus on what matters most in the long run-- — working on your inside physical and emotional well being.

Part Five

How Far?

Fear motivation comes from being scared of losing something valuable. Fear will motivate you in the beginning, yet it cannot be very rewarding or long-lasting. It will not sustain you.

Greg Ryan

9

Voices in Your Head

In the movie "Forest Gump" Forest was encouraged his hole childhood to, *"Run Forest Run."* One day as an adult he decides to do just that. He runs, runs and run some more. After going clear across the country he decides, just as fast as he started to stop. *"I'm through runnin now,"* he says. Turns around and walks back the way he came; a sudden drastic change of heart to say the least. Do you think Forest was running from his fear of inadequacy or because people admired him, or both?

Not quit sure why Forest started running, but I think he stops running out of a revelation in his head. He finally realizes that no matter how far he goes the voices still would still be there; never able to out run them. The pleasurable feeling of being noticed was not as big as the fear of not measuring up; in the end the motivation to continue ran out.

Are you like Forest Gump? How many miles are you going to put between the reality of your health and the voices in your head, only to realize they're still there, stronger than ever? How far will you go out of fear, how far will you travel to seek pleasure and peace? How long will you listen to the voices in your head?

While this is not a psychology book the truth is, it's your emotions that are dictating your health; maybe even more so than the physical. Think about it!

10
Fear Runner to Pleasure Seeker

How am I motivated? How far will I let this go?

? What will it take to get you started? What will keep you going in down times?

No matter how hard you try, how many self-help books you buy, you just cannot seem to get or stay motivated. Why?

Most people think they are motivated, and they may very well be, in the short term, but eventually for most the gas runs out. Two main emotions push people to exercise: FEAR AND/OR PLEASURE.

It is important to know how you are motivated in order to keep on track for the long haul. Connecting the two, the mind and body--with your spirit makes all the difference in the world and really is the most important aspect of any successful fitness program.

Fear Runners

Fear the most powerful motivator pushes people to do things that normally they may not every think of doing. You may get motivated to exercise because you are afraid of the consequences of aging, getting a disease, developing cancer or even dying. You run from the reality. If this is how YOU are motivated you are a FEAR RUNNER.

Fear can be a very powerful force to get things accomplished or just the opposite nothing done. Being motivated by fear is ok in the short term, but sooner or later it's not very rewarding to the soul. What do you do when something doesn't satisfy; you either quit doing it or turn to something else?

Most individuals start exercise programs out of fear which is ok, but in the end the benefits must out weigh the fear in order to be fore filled. What ever it takes in the beginning to get you started, I say.

Pleasure Seekers

Let's be real, exercise can hurt and most of the time is uncomfortable at best. However, you feel rejuvenated, stronger, more confident and healthier after you've done it. You receive emotional pleasure. Striving to seek pleasure through exercise can be much more motivating and enlightening in the end.

Fear Runner to a Pleasure Seeker

The goal is to sustain your motivation for the long-term and to develop a lifestyle that reflects good health. It should also be a goal to make it halfway fun; turning your desires from fear into desires of pleasure.

In a perfect world what works well is to have a small amount of fear (not take life for granted) and a lot of pleasure motivation (wanting to feel better badly).

For example, you might be motivated because you fear your blood pressure will get to high, but you're also motivated by how much better you feel after you exercise; both a fear and pleasure motivation. Whatever the combination may be make sure fear is not the dominating emotion in the end. Being motivated by pleasure will take you much further toward your goal of being healthier.

11
A Change of Heart

How do I know what my desire to exercise is?

Having a desire is much more powerful than being motivated. The desire fuels the motives and usually comes from two emotional sources: *Extrinsic or Intrinsic.*

Outside or Extrinsic Desires

Having a flat stomach, thin hips, lean muscular arms and a physically fit look are big motivators; while great in the short-term this is not what you want your overall reward to be. If your main desire is to look better and improve outward appearance, it probably means you are headed for disappointment due to aging.

Inside or Intrinsic Desires

The desire to exercise needs to come from *inside* your body; your reasons are centered on lowering your blood pressure, leveling cholesterol, getting more energy, losing excess weight and toning up. Having internal desires to exercise and eat better will prove more rewarding in the long-term.

A Change of Heart

A change in attitude takes place for most people in their forties; reality sets in. We want to look twenty-five again, but we know deep down it will never see those years again. What you need is a change of heart!

Your thought process must change from external to internal. In other words, start focusing on the bigger picture. Concentrate on better energy levels, our body's vital signs such as cholesterol — triglyceride levels, blood pressure, and body fat measurements.

When you focus and improve on these and a host of other aspects of health, the visual improvements are perks the program.

12
Effortless Benefits

How and when do my desires become habitual?

 Exercise becomes a habit when the benefits outweigh the effort. If your thinking is always on how much effort it takes or how discomforting the active is you will always find a reason not to get exercise.

The truth is you may never thoroughly enjoy exercising, but you may learn to look forward to the benefits of doing it. Some are immediate feel-good emotions: others are long-term vital signs, energy levels, and better overall health.

Whatever the benefits are you have a better chance of sticking to an exercise program if you have experienced *"the highs."* If you learn to associate the good feelings with exercise you will find yourself exercising more consistently. On the other hand, if you continually focus on the effort it takes to exercise, the time and the discomfort, you may very well talk yourself out of it. Bottom line, the benefits outweigh the effort many times over.

Point of no return

Growing up I was an introvert with a low self-esteem. However, through the emotional power of exercise and eating well, I developed a change of heart over time.

Today I am both fear-motivated and pleasure-driven; fear in the sense that I don't take anything for granted and pleasure in the fact that I look forward to the confidence after exercise.

Quite frankly, I have no desire to go back to the old person I once was, nor can I not afford emotionally to go back. I must go forward, day-by-day, workout-by-workout, and meal-by-meal.

Honestly, I can't imagine the rest of my life without exercise or good eating habits. It truly has become effortless!

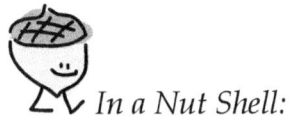 *In a Nut Shell:*

How Far are you going to let your health decline? How long are you going to hide behind the illusions in your head? That's right,

Are you willing to look at changing your fitness for the long haul or are you one of those wishful short-term try- it-and-see
people?

Are you willing to have a change in attitude toward aging? Are you willing to look at the benefits of exercise and eating rather than resenting the painful effort you think it will take to get there?

How far are you willing to go and risk everything.

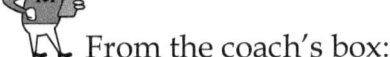 From the coach's box:

➢ Establish what makes you tick. How are you are motivated most of the time?

- ➢ Use both fear and pleasure to motivate you to move forward.

- ➢ Focus on the benefits of exercise and eat right for more emotional rewards.

- ➢ Get past the point of no return. When you miss the benefits and feelings that go along with fitness, you will be more likely to continue.

Part Six

What For?

A broken bone.........................$10,000
Open heart surgery...............$100,000
Nursing home care – Yearly.....$36,000

Daily exercise.....................Priceless

13
Just One....

"Please, please just give me one more, I'll never ask again!"

Have you every asked, prayed, or pleaded for just one more of something; one more chance, opportunity, or day to make it right?

When my dad was in the hospital a few years ago, I prayed that I would be able to have one more day with him, one more opportunity to go fishing, one additional moment in time to say, I love you. I was blessed to have that chance, yesterday I was not.

"Have you seen Jim lately?" I asked as we got to the first tee. *"Greg, he died two months ago."*
"You're kidding, right?"
"No Melanoma got him pretty quickly."

In a million years I never thought Jim would die so young, especially like that.

All I could think about was how we left it; how I left it. Oh, I wish I had just one more basketball game with him, one more night out with the guys, one more "See you tomorrow, Jim."

Boy, what I would give to not have left our relationship the way I did. If only I had known.

14
For Who?

For You

Why should I exercise? You owe it to yourself. For once in your life, **you can be selfish** and not feel guilty. It's your body and your heart; why not take better care of it?

There will never be enough time or the right moment to begin. So why not start today, for your benefit? With no illusions of perfection and no unattainable expectations, the ride can be an enjoyable one. It doesn't have to be from resentment, pride, or comparisons. Don't let life pass you by. Get on board now!

For Others

If taking better care of your self isn't a powerful enough reason to get you started exercising, maybe you could start by doing it for someone you care about.

How about being a good example for your kids or your spouse maybe would like to have a more relaxed person around? Don't you want to be around to enjoy life with the ones you love?

For Country

Diabetes and health care will cost America one hundred twenty-two billion dollars this year alone. You can help not pass on that cost on to others and your children tomorrow by doing something today.

15
Personally Yours
(unedited)

Stubbornness; that's all I can say. Today I learned that my friend Jim's the latest of many people I've known over the years that I've tried and tried to reach out to; only to be squashed by pride and denial. Now they've fallen; fallen into a hole they will never get out of, death and destruction.

It breaks my heart to see their family's go through this. It frustrates me to no end to know that their end could have turned out much, much different. It makes me mad as heck to know that your personal hang-ups will cost you dearly someday. I, rather than some doctor tries to explain to you that you need to get some exercise and eat better, but what do you do, you go on your marry way with all the lame excuses not to take some action?

Why? Because you're afraid of failing, what friend's might say, you're not worthy enough or it won't happen to me; give me a break people.

No, these words aren't politically correct, but I just don't care anymore. Why, because you're dying inside and out? You want to die a slow death, go ahead. You want to live the remaining days of your life depressed, cynical and in fear, go ahead. It's personally your choice.

The problem is I do care; I care too much about you living a more fore filled life. I care that there are more obese people now than over weight. I care that half of you will get or have diabetes. I care that your kids won't live past your age now. I care that one out of three of you will break a bone. I care that most of you are depressed and suffer from low self-esteem. I care that you're getting older and physically feeling more miserable by the day.

Personally, your choices today are life and death related. The truth is, you probably don't want to deal with them, its' just too painful (so you think). Today, I'm begging you to come to your senses. Today, I'm asking you to take a personal stake in your health. Today, I'm going out of a limb to tell you how I really feel about your health. Today, I don't care if you like me or read another word of in my books. Today, I lay it all of the line; truth or the consequences, which one will it be? Personally Yours,

Gregory Patrick Ryan

Addendum

As an extra bonus I would like to share with you how I have kept my body-fat down all these years.

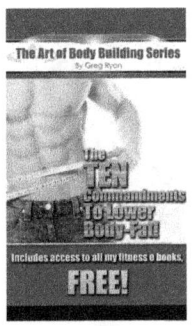

I have kept my body-fat lower than fourteen percent for almost thirty years. This may not sound so remarkable to you, but to me it's been a life saver. You don't know it, but my family is full of diabetes, obesity, heart disease, depression and for one to beat those odds for so long, is not easy. However, this was not always so! It has been a struggle to say the least.

Fat Little Kids

I grew up with very little self-esteem or respect for my health. As a farm boy you have a built in activity regiment in daily farm chores, but that's as far as the exercise went. There's a difference between having to do something and wanting to. I just didn't want to do anything.

Fitness found me over time and so did a certain attitude that I would like to share in the next few pages. For what ever reason from day one in the gym I believed a persons body-fat levels were true indicators of fitness. I also believed as a true body builder keeping your body-fat levels low as possible through the off seasons and year round was the ultimate. Any one can gain size, weight and even muscle, but not everyone can have the ideal balance of muscle to fat year after year; but I made a decision early on to try, and boy I'm glad I did.

Why you should read this e book!

This e book is not like most articles on health, fitness and even body-fat. This book is solely based off of my experience over the last thirty years and what worked for me.

Any guy can put on muscle size and any woman can get thin, but few can get their body-fat levels low and maintain it.

Contents

Introduction

Too many people focus on the scale, and in the end lose the battle mentally and physically. If you pants are lose, muscles defined and tight, why do you care what the scale registers? Any body can lose or gain weight, but a much less percentage of people keep their body-fat at a respectable level. And very few can maintain it lower than normal for years, I did.

No matter what your age, keeping a lower level of body-fat is vital. If you are of the younger generation then you look better if you are a baby boomer or older a lower fat level is an extremely healthier state of being. This e book outlines just a few ways I have kept my body-fat low for many years. Don't be fooled by the length or lack of gimmicky phrases, its straight for and proven.

There is no magic formula, but there are a few things that will make the process easier.

Part 1
Mental Body-Fat

"Losing body-fat may be just as much mental as physical!"

I
Balance

"You have to constantly juggle your mind and body to lower-body fat!"

Solving the whole body-fat thing can be summed up in one word, *"Balance;"* a much easy word to write than to succeed, I must say.

Balance- *"An equality between the sums total of the two sides."* In fitness and body-fat there are a few more sides of the equation than just two.

Never Ending Challenge

I was not in a very good mood yesterday and I stated the following to one of my clients, *"If you think for one second that you will work really hard, reach a goal and all will be perfect, you are sorely mistaken and will in the end be very disappointed."*

The same attitude must apply to acquiring an ideal body fat level over time. You must take a life long, day to day approach. Balancing anything in life is usually the biggest challenge any of us will every have. Add the balancing of the ideal workout and eating plan to normal life and it can be doubly as challenging.

The Approach

When I first started workout I had ZERO discipline, faith in myself or confidence that I would or could succeed. Fortunately for some reason I just believed this, *"If I could just get through one day, and one day only at a time then I would worry about tomorrow, well, tomorrow."*

The Attitude

Not to jump ahead but I also learned over time that having a balanced workout, eating and life plan all the time was pretty much impossible. When one area of the plan is doing well, you have to shift gears to another area. When that one is under control then either the first one or another totally different area of your life and fitness plan needs to be worked on.

My point is this, the goal to lower your body fat is to achieve as close to a balanced plan of all the important things as one possibly can. However, you need to understand that you will never get it perfect, nor if you think you have it, then it will not take long before an area needs more tweaking. You will always be seeking a balanced approach to fitness. The closer you get to it, and the longer you can achieve it, the lower your body-fat will go and stay.

The Area's

There are three main areas I want to focus on in this e book. Each one does not work with out the other. Like a spoke in a wheel with out one the tire will go flat; so goes your body-fat. The three main areas are: <u>Psychology,</u> <u>Nutrition</u> and <u>Physical Training</u>.

Again, allow me to challenge you to take a long term approach, and an attitude that each day will be a constant balancing act of all three areas.

II
Body vs. Mind

"Lowering body-fat takes more faith at times than fitness!"

While a balanced approach is the key, I never said it would be easy. Maintaining the momentum and synergy of everything may come down to more mental than physical. The challenge with the whole subject of body-fat is we can't see it totally. You can look good, but still have less than desirable body-fat levels. The goal is to keep the EGO in check; easier said than done.

Mirrors and Clothes Don't Lie

Man or woman it doesn't matter the mind and EGO is an internal competitor; for woman its vanity, for men it's about being moncho. You can very easily get off base by focusing too much on looks, or bench press numbers, rather than the levels of fat you have.

I've always tried to express to people that at the end of the day, the mirror and clothes don't lie; meaning those two things probably are more accurate of your over all health than a scale.

Chances are if your clothes are feeling loser then your body-fat is most likely decreasing; not always though.

What you can't see may kill you

Diabetes is one of the fastest growing diseases today. On some level it seems as though you wake up one morning and you have it; that's really not the case. Developing Diabetes is a process that takes time. Poor eating habits, lack of exercise and genetics all contribute to such a disease. Not being able to see the development of diabetes in our bodies makes us not take it so serious or even increase a state of denial.

The chance's of getting diabetes in your body has been there for some time, but it was not visual so it never crossed your mind. One morning you awake and the doctor says, "Yep, you got it." Diabetes is caused by high levels of body-fat by the way.

You take a similar approach to your body-fat levels, if you can't see it then you assume it's not a problem, or worse yet, not even on the radar screen of life.

Body Fat-Thin is NOT In

Thin is NOT in! When I worked for Kathy Smith in Los Angeles, California I managed about fifty employees; ten of them were aerobic instructors.

Out of the ten half weighed an average of 115 pounds. The shocking thing was come to find out through a club testing day most of them were clinically considered obese. What? How can that be? By looking at them you would draw the conclusion that they were in great shape; and to the public eye they were.

Thin is NOT In

The tests discovered that over thirty percent of their total body weight was in the form of fat, medically, making them fit into the obese category; totally shocking to the naked eye. So be very careful not to distort the idea that thinness equals healthiness.

In short for the instructors, to high heart rate over time ate away at muscle tissue, combined with poor eating habits eventually made their ratio of muscle to overall body weight out of balance.

Contrast this with some football players who are big and bulky and the same thing occurs, too much weight and a decrease in muscle can make you obese with out looking like it.

Part 2
Physical Body-Fat

"Understanding what body-fat is and the importance of lowering it is half the battle!"

III
Body-Fat

"Getting muscular or losing weight is one thing, lowering your body-fat is another story!"

What is Body-Fat?

Body fat is a compound comprised of glycerol -- a substance formed in fatty acids -- and fatty acids which is required as a concentrated energy source for our muscles. Fat is a storage substance for the body's extra calories and it fills fat cells (adipose tissue) that help insulate the body. When the body has used up the calories from carbohydrates it begins to depend on the calories from fat.

How can I determine body fat percentage?

There are several ways to find out your body fat percentage. Unfortunately, the more accurate the method, the more of a hassle and/or expensive it tends to be.

DEXA scan – full body X-ray scan of the same type used for bone density. Very accurate.

Hydrostatic Weighing – Weighing under water (completely submerged, with all air blown out of lungs) – Very accurate when done professionally.

Skin-fold calipers ("pinch test") – Simple, but needs to be done by someone who is trained, and you can't do it on yourself. Wide variations in accuracy for people without training.

Bioelectrical Impedance (BIA) – These are scales and hand-held devises that run low-level (and painless) electrical current through you. They can be accurate, although the accuracy varies according to the specific device (do your research) and how it is used.

Best results are obtained first thing in the morning with no alcohol consumed for 2 days prior, and no exercise the night before.

Navy tape measure method - This is a formula based on several body measurements taken with a tape measure. It can be quite accurate (it is used by the military), but it does depend upon your ability to accurately measure. Using centimeters rather than inches is the best, but using inches within ¼ of an inch works. To be sure, measure yourself 3 times and take the average.

What's the difference between Body Fat Percentage and BMI?

BMI (body mass index) is a formula based on height and weight. It was developed because in the general population, it is correlated with body fat. However, there are quite a few groups of people for whom BMI is not as accurate -- short women and muscular people, to name two.

BMI also varies according to some ethnic groups. Also, for people who are interested in changing their body composition and not just their weight, knowing body fat percentage is an improvement over BMI. For example, if you are exercising to build muscle (a good goal), knowing your body fat percentage is a good idea.

Also, when losing weight, you want to preserve as much lean body mass as possible. (Low-carb diets generally produce better results than high carb ones for this purpose.)

If you want to lose or gain weight, you need to be able to measure the state your body is in now and then monitor the changes as you add or subtract calories from your diet. One way to do this is to calculate and monitor your Body Mass Index (BMI).

Since a typical scale only measures your total weight, it helps to have more information to determine if that weight is healthy or unhealthy. A person who is six feet tall and weighs 198 pounds is probably going to have a smaller amount of body fat than a person who is five feet tall and 198 pounds.

The BMI combines your weight and your height into a score that helps you determine if you are underweight, at a healthy weight, overweight, or obese.

BMI is calculated with the following formula:

weight (lb) / [height (in)]^2 x 703 or in

metric:weight (kg) / [height (m)]^2

What Your BMI Means

You can compare your BMI to this table to help you determine whether you're at a healthy weight.

- Underweight = less than 18.5

- Normal weight = 18.5-24.9

- Overweight = 25-29.9

- Obese = 30 or greater

If you are planning to lose or gain weight, you can use your BMI to monitor your progress. It's important to know that your BMI is not the same as your body fat percentage, which is a different number and doesn't correspond to these charts.

People who have a BMI in the overweight or obese ranges may have a higher risk of cardiovascular disease, diabetes, arthritis, and some forms of cancer. However, it's important to see your health care provider, who can take other lifestyle and risk factors into consideration.

The BMI isn't perfect because it's an indirect measurement of fat, and really doesn't differentiate pounds of fat from pounds of muscle and bone. So it doesn't work well for very muscular people or for people who have lost a lot of muscle mass.

For example, an elite athlete with a very small amount of body fat will still have a high BMI, and an elderly person may have a lower BMI because they have less muscle mass. In these cases, a better method of measurement is the body fat percentage.

By the Numbers

If you are a numbers person here are ones to shoot for when trying to lower your body fat.

Age	Under fat	Healthy Range	Overweight	Obese
20-40 yrs	Under 21%	21-33%	33-39%	Over 39%
41-60 yrs	Under 23%	23-35%	35-40%	Over 40%
61-79 yrs	Under 24%	24-36%	36-42%	Over 42%

Men

Age	Under fat	Healthy Range	Overweight	Obese
20-40 yrs	Under 8%	8-19%	19-25%	Over 25%
41-60 yrs	Under 11%	11-22%	22-27%	Over 27%
61-79 yrs	Under 13%	13-25%	25-30%	Over 30%

Above Average Below Grade

Unfortunately most of you are above the average, and in the body-fat category anything above is not good. So what grade will you give yourself?

There are many things that contribute to higher body-fat but in this book we will only concentrate on a few of the things that will give you more bang for the buck. For me there a few major things that I concentrated on daily that helped me keep my body-fat low for years.

IV
Blood Sugar

"Blood Sugar, Food and Training- The Ultimate Goal!"

For the last twenty five years or so I have had one daily goal. I found by achieving this goal each day, my body-fat would stay at a lower level. I understood that if I monitored and regulated my blood sugar levels through good nutritional habits, and a balanced exercise program the rest would kind of fall into place.

What is Blood Sugar?

In short, blood **sugar** concentration or blood glucose level **is** the amount of glucose (**sugar**) present in the blood.

Blood sugar, also known as blood glucose, is the body's fuel that feeds the brain, nervous system, and tissues. A healthy body makes glucose not only from ingested carbohydrates, but also from proteins and fats, and would not be able to function without it. Maintaining a balanced blood glucose level is essential to a body's everyday performance.

Glucose is absorbed directly into the bloodstream from the intestine and results in a rapid increase in the blood glucose level. The pancreas releases insulin, a natural hormone, to prevent blood glucose levels from excessively elevating, and aids in the moving of glucose into the cells. Glucose is then carried to each cell, providing them with the energy needed to carry out its specific function.

Healthy blood glucose levels are considered to be in the 70-120 range. One high or low reading does not always indicate a problem, but the glucose level should be monitored for 10-14 days. There are several different tests that can be administered to determine whether an individual has a problem maintaining a normal glucose level such as: a fasting blood sugar test, an oral glucose test, or a random blood sugar test. Blood glucose levels that remain either too high or too low over time, may cause damage to the eyes, kidneys, nerves and blood vessels.

Hypoglycemia

Hypoglycemia is a condition caused by low blood sugar levels in the body, can be extremely debilitating if not controlled properly. Symptoms include shaking, irritability, confusion, strange behavior and even loss of consciousness. These symptoms can be corrected by ingesting a form of a sugar such as a hard candy, a sugar pill, or a sweet drink. Ingesting one or more of these forms of sugar quickly raises the body's blood sugar level and has an almost immediate effect.

Hyperglycemia

Hyperglycemia occurs when the blood glucose levels in the body are higher than normal. Symptoms of this condition include: excessive thirst, frequent urination, tiredness, weakness and lethargy. If the levels become excessively high, a person can become dehydrated and comatose.

A Side Note

Diabetes occurs when the pancreas either produces little or no insulin, or the cells do not respond appropriately to the insulin produced. There are three main types of diabetes: Type 1 , Type 2, and Gestational Diabetes. Type 1 diabetes occurs when the body's immune system attacks insulin producing cells in the pancreas destroying them and causing the pancreas to produce little or no insulin. Type 2 diabetes is the most common and is associated with age, obesity, and genetics. Gestational diabetes develops only during pregnancy, but means an increase in the chance of the woman developing Type 2 diabetes in the future. All types of diabetes are serious and need to be monitored regularly.

Insulin Resistance

What is insulin resistance?

Insulin resistance is a condition in which the body produces insulin but does not use it properly. Insulin, a hormone made by the pancreas, helps the body use glucose for energy. Glucose is a form of sugar that is the body's main source of energy.

The body's digestive system breaks food down into glucose, which then travels in the bloodstream to cells throughout the body. Glucose in the blood is called blood glucose, also known as blood sugar. As the blood glucose level rises after a meal, the pancreas releases insulin to help cells take in and use the glucose.

When people are insulin resistant, their muscle, fat, and liver cells do not respond properly to insulin. As a result, their bodies need more insulin to help glucose enter cells. The pancreas tries to keep up with this increased demand for insulin by producing more. Eventually, the pancreas fails to keep up with the body's need for insulin.

Excess glucose builds up in the bloodstream, setting the stage for diabetes. Many people with insulin resistance have high levels of both glucose and insulin circulating in their blood at the same time.

Insulin resistance increases the chance of developing type 2 diabetes and heart disease. Learning about insulin resistance is the first step toward making lifestyle changes that can help prevent diabetes and other health problems.

What causes insulin resistance?

Scientists have identified specific genes that make people more likely to develop insulin resistance and diabetes. Excess weight and lack of physical activity also contribute to insulin resistance.

Many people with insulin resistance and high blood glucose have other conditions that increase the risk of developing type 2 diabetes and damage to the heart and blood vessels, also called cardiovascular disease.

These conditions include having excess weight around the waist, high blood pressure, and abnormal levels of cholesterol and triglycerides in the blood. Having several of these problems is called metabolic syndrome or insulin resistance syndrome, formerly called syndrome X.

Roller (coaster)

A good indicator (or one for me) that my blood sugar levels were off during the day was my tiredness around mid morning and afternoon.

If you look at roller coasters you will basically find two kinds; hilly ones and those that just go straight up and down. Or maybe we could visualize a one hump camel or a two humped one. Either way, the goals is to not have too many humps (ups and downs) in your blood sugar levels through out the day.

Two Humped Camels

When your blood sugar levels, or energy levels go up and down like a two humped camel you

DO NOT burn body-fat. Chances are you will probably do the opposite of what you should do. (See the nutritional chapter)

The Five Hour Energy Craze

Each year American's consume about eight hundred million dollars of the product called, "Five Hour Energy Drink." Why, because, most people are tired either mid morning or mid afternoon? The drink apparently revives you long enough (five hours) to get through the rest of your day. All it is, is caffeine and mineral water. The company is basically making boat loads of money off of people's LAZINESS.

I really believe that people's biggest problem of obesity and high body-fat levels is due to poor regulation of their blood sugars caused by lack of exercise and poor eating habits.

Blood Sugar Regulation

Blood sugar levels are regulated by negative feedback in order to keep the body in homeostasis.

The levels of glucose in the blood are monitored by the cells in the pancreas's Islets of Langerhans.

If the blood glucose level falls to dangerous levels (as in very heavy exercise or lack of food for extended periods), the Alpha cells of the pancreas release glucagon, a hormone whose effects on liver cells act to increase blood glucose levels. They convert glycogen into glucose (this process is called glycogenolysis). The glucose is released into the bloodstream, increasing blood sugar levels.

While far as I know I am not diabetic or even pre-diabetic, however for me the whole ball of wax came down to, *"HOW do I control and regulate my blood sugar levels every single day?"* It came down to two categories; eating and exercising smart.

Here are a few ways I regulated by blood sugar levels:

- Eat often
- Never skip breakfast
- Don't eat past 8 at night
- No white flour at noon or evening meals
- Protein snacks between meals
- Workout in the morning

Part 3
Consumable Body-Fat

"Balance the diet and solve your body-fat issue, half way!"

V
Binging- Portion Control

"Control the roller coaster and cure the body-fat!"

Call it any thing you want, but eating to much food in too little time in my mind is binging; and binging cause blood sugar problems which in the long run raises body-fat levels.

If you really want to know how much you are eating, just calculate all the calories you consume in a day, or in each meal at the very least. I would be willing to bet you would be surprised and even shocked at the amount of calories consumed or inhaled.

You always hear about snacking and eating smaller meals through out the day, why? By nature we eat more when we eat less often.

One feeds on the other

We talked about blood sugar levels and the important of keeping them even through out the day, but it also must be noted how low blood sugar levels promote bigger portion sizes, in turn larger portion sizes spike blood sugar levels and then they crash. Each one feeds on the other building up so much momentum that in some cases if you don't exercise you run the risk of becoming pre-diabetic or worse full blown diabetes.

VI
Before Noon
"Early bird gets the energy"

If I have any secrets to keeping my body fat lower than most here's one of them; I front load my carbohydrates daily.

Carbohydrate FRONT Loading

What the heck do you mean Front loading your carbohydrates?

Let's look at the habits of most people. One reason so many people have gotten fatter over the years is because of convenience, laziness and lack of planning their foods. What food group is the easiest to get and fix? Yes, carbohydrates. And when do people eat the majority of those carbohydrates, at night, right? What do carbohydrates supply to the body? Yes, energy. When do we need the most energy, at night or in the morning? So, what's wrong with this picture then?

Eating good food can still make you fat

In the early nineties a study came out on how good pasta was for you, so what did people do? They ate more pasta.

American's are almost twenty percent fatter today than back then. How can that be, pasta was suppose to be good for you? It is, however, consumed at night followed by a night on your back, converts into glucose and over time, fat.

Front Loading

You hear of carbohydrate loading in sports so I guess you could say that I carbohydrates loaded to keep my body-fat low. Well a better and more accurate way of saying it is, I FRONT loaded my carbohydrate intake. In other words, if I want to keep my body-fat lower I will eat the majority of my carbohydrates, more importantly the complex carbs prior to the two o'clock hour.

Part 4
Training to Lower Body-Fat

"Physical exercise is like a tool of a sculpture, if used just enough, art is created!"

VII
Beliefs from the Core

"Having a little faith may be the most important action to lower body-fat!"

The core muscle groups may be the most functional and important muscle groups in your body. They also may be the most neglected out of them all as well.

Your Belief System

One thing I learned early on in my body building career was that you have to have a strong belief in working out your core muscles. It's very easy to make any excuse NOT to exercise the core muscles.

The other thing is, they HURT. Doing core muscle group exercises are painful, so you have to believe in what you are doing at the time, a little faith goes along ways.

Faith

Having faith in something you can't see is challenging to say the least. Just looking at your body in the mirror is no accurate way of measuring body-fat. You can't even muster a good guess by a visual.

VIII
Blood Work

In the beginning chapter of this book we discussed the importance of being balanced. When it comes to physical training to lower your body-fat it's a dicey path. It really is a balancing act of good food, sleep, a stress free attitude, cardiovascular and strength training. The goal is to rid the body of fat while at the same time continue to develop lean muscle tissue.

Blood Flow- Cardiovascular Training

Just walking, biking, crossfit or step class does not cut it when it comes to losing weight and body-fat. I can not remember the last I went into a gym and saw a member check their heart rate zone.

Target Heart Rate Zone

There is no way you will get to your ideal body-fat weight unless you hit your target heart rate zone every time you perform cardiovascular training; don't go over or under, you have to hit the target.

If you go over you burn valuable muscle, under and weight stays on. Memorize this formula;

220-age x 60-85% = Target Heart Rate (THR)

Cardiovascular Training Protocol

Like I said, I never see people take their heart rates, machine or by hand. So here is the protocol you should follow to lower the fat levels efficiently:

1. First and fore most calculate your heart rate numbers. You only have to do this once and memorize the zone and divide by six.
2. No matter what cardiovascular piece of equipment you use by the seven minute mark of your workout you should and must be in your zone. Most people are not in there until twelve to fifteen minutes in.
3. Maintain this zone for a minimum of twenty minutes and a maximum of forty minutes.

4. Don't just get off of the equipment at the end, slow the pace down gradually; this is the cool-down period. Cardiac arrest may occur if you don't cool down properly.

Cannibalism

Cannibals eat their own. If you exercise with your heart rate to high your muscles eat their own.

The average weight of my aerobic instructors in LA was around 115 pounds. After a surprise body-fat test, over half were clinically obese. How is that possible? Cannibalism!

Day after day they failed to monitor their heart rates, thus they were too high. Day after day their bodies were not being fueled properly for their training regiment. With the combination of the two, their body's recuperation process could not keep up with the demand they had been putting on themselves.

Over time, precious muscle tissue was being eaten away like hungry, desperate pack man. Eventually, the percentage of body-fat to their over all weight was close or over thirty percent, clinically obese numbers. Ouch!

More is not better either!

Don't make the mistake of trying to put logic with exercise, your dealing with a human body that in the end will not be able to totally manipulate. Those aerobic instructors for some reason thought that the more they did, the higher they kept their heart rates the less they would weight and lower the body-fat. Unfortunately, all that did was hurt their health not help it.

Cycle Intensity Levels

Adaptation is a word you will hear me say frequently. I truly believe the body is smart and has a good memory. This will take some pre-planning on your part, however, maybe one of the smartest and most effective techniques I have used in keeping my body-fat low over the years.

In other words, never do the same identical cardiovascular workout three times in a row. This can be accomplished by changing length of workouts, elevations or intensity levels, time during the day or even locations.

IX
Body Work

Cardiovascular is aerobic and weight training is anaerobic, we all know this, however, there is one little thing I have discovered over the years when it comes to weight training and body-fat.

We are all taught as well as you have learned in this book that a combination of food, cardiovascular and now weight training aids in lowering body-fat. Now let's dissect this theory a little bit more in detail as it pertains to weight training and body-fat.

Flipping the Switch

I truly believe that you can keep your body-fat lower over time more so than even most people imagine as it pertains to weights. Not so much the exercises, but the technique in which you go through the workouts. Over the years I learned to flip a switch right before I walked into the gym.

Time Lines

The first thing I did was, decide to put a time limit to my weight training workouts.
Whether I was done with my body-parts or not I would walk out of the gym. Walking out once or twice cured me of messing around.

The Art of Flow

I have been complimented time and time again for how artful my workouts look. From afar there seems to be a sense of methodical flow from rep to set, exercise to machine; an effortless motion. Like I mentioned, flipping the mental switch and times lines cut my time down between sets and exercises and in the long run by doing this my body-fat stayed lower.

Call it, flow, intensity, focus what ever you want to, all I know is, body-fat stayed off, I had more fun and received more results in a shorter period of time.

X
Bonus

Variety

I am convinced that our bodies get bored with what we do physically, adapt and plateau in getting results. Mentally we get stale and that translates into physical stagnation. Then what do you do? You quit.

Pre Planning

Putting variety into your workouts and eating habits takes a little thinking ahead; this is why most don't do it, its too much work. However, pre-planning your workouts and eating accomplishes two things, takes a lot of wasted energy and time out of your life and builds confidence, which in turn creates momentum.

Workout Variety

Our bodies start getting use to repetitive actions with in our workouts around six to eight weeks into a workout plan.

I really can not explain it, but the body assumes you are going to do the same exercise, weight and order of those exercises after a certain time. When this happens the body plateaus and in some cases the body fat goes up, because the heart rate stays at a lower rate through out the workout.

Food Variety

Maybe it's the typical number of calories, I'm not sure but just as with a typical workout for you the body gets use to the same old foods you eat as well. If you have oatmeal and wheat toast every morning for breakfast even though the food types are good for you the calorie amount stays the same. Over time the body gets use to that amount of calories and again, the metabolism slows down.

Conclusion

For overall health stand point, there is nothing more valuable than keeping your body-fat in check. If you are concerned about appearance, a body never looks better than lean and mean. Achieving such a goal is not as hard as *keeping* ones body-fat lower; it really does take a *balanced* approach.

In my opinion, it's easy to put on muscle or lose weight, but it's much more difficult to do both at the same time; its quality not quantity. Quality muscle and low body mass takes a juggling act on a consistent basis and in the end it maybe more of a *mind* game than anything.

In order to over come something you have to understand what it is and why its there. Body-fat is not Body Mass. Body-fat is not necessarily pounds read on a scale either.

Remember to keep the first things first, and always focus on *blood sugar*. If you regulate your blood sugar the body-fat has to stay low. I realize life is hectic these days, however some way some how you have to *pre plan*, set goals and be proactive verses reactive. If you don't, you will constantly eat more than you should, throwing your metabolism into a free fall.

Body-fat tends to come off easier when the metabolism stays constant through out the day not the evening so watch those high energy foods late at night. You have to realize that it's not all about exercise, it's about food too. But when you do exercise more is NOT better. Be smart, efficient and precise. Monitor your efforts, structure with variety works best for me. You do all this one day you will awake and guess what, the switch is flipped and the body-fat has gone.

Its not rocket science, but it will take work. And I know you've heard this a lot, but seriously, if I've done this you can too; one goal, one day, one meal, one workout, one percent body-fat at a time.

Good Luck!

For FREE Fitness Advice go here
Blogs:
www.resolutionsblog.com
www.reso-care.com
www.gregryanfitness.com

 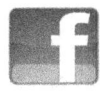 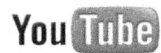 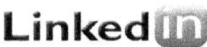

Check out my entire book collection at

   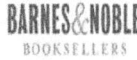